VITAMIN DEFICIENCIES

Table of Content:

Chapter 1 General

The study of thiamine deficiency earned its author the Nobel Prize (Eijkman 1929). The research connected with vitamin C was likewise awarded this prestigious prize (Haworth and Szent-Gyorgyi, 1937). Below we briefly discuss several selected hypovitaminoses that may pose problems in clinical practice. Certain chapters (e.g. folic acid deficiency, iodine deficiency, ...) were not completed on time for this CD and will be incorporated in an updated version at a later date.

Chapter 2 Beriberi

2.1 Beriberi, Summary

- Thiamine = vitamin B1, water-soluble, heat-labile
- Deficiency caused by either lack of thiamine intake or destruction by thiaminases.
- Symptoms may develop acutely.
- Dry beriberi: neuritis with paralysis and loss of sensation.
- Wet beriberi: high-output heart failure.
- Cerebral beriberi: ocular motility disorders, mental confusion, ataxia.
- Infantile beriberi: aphonia, areflexia and heart failure.

2.2 Beriberi, Thiamine - General

Vitamin B1, or thiamine, is a water-soluble, heat-sensitive vitamin which is present in many foods: meat, grain products, potatoes, beans, nuts and yeast. The refining of sugar, rice and grain products reduces the thiamine content. The polishing of brown rice (removal of the dry outer layer) reduces the content of vitamin B1 to practically zero. Thiamine is destroyed during food preparation by prolonged heating or is often washed away with the cooking water. Some nutrients contain thiaminases which have the ability to break down vitamin B1 in the food: raw fish, coffee and tea. Certain plants contain thiaminases and are consequently toxic. The uptake of thiamine takes place in the proximal small intestine. A small amount is stored in muscle tissue. Vitamin B1 is an important component of enzymes of carbohydrate metabolism (decarboxylation of alpha- keto acids). Thiamine pyrophosphate is the active co-enzyme of transketolase, an enzyme of the pentose monophosphates shunt (carbohydrate metabolism). Thiamine is important for neural cell membranes and it has a modulating function in neuromuscular transmission.

2.3 Beriberi, Historical Overview

At the end of the 16th century, the first reports emerged of a new disorder in the Far East. In Indonesia this disease was called beriberi. The etymology of the word is not clear. Dr Jacobus Bontius reported that beriberi is similar to the local name for sheep, and was believed to refer to the peculiar gait of that animal. Together with Nicolas Tulp from Holland (cf. the painting "The Anatomy Lesson of Dr Tulp" by Rembrandt, 1632) he gave the first European description of the disease. In Hindi, the term „bharbari" means swelling; in Arabic the term „burh" means shortness of breath; and „bahri" means marine. In Singhalese, „bhayree" means weakness. Beriberi was found to be a ravaging disease which occurred with varying frequency. This was dramatically illustrated in 1883 when a training ship of the Japanese navy sailed to New Zealand. Of the crew of 278 sailors and officer cadets, 161 fell ill with beriberi and 25 died of the disease. On the recommendation of the Japanese medical officer Takaki, a different diet was used, with more milk, condensed milk, bread and vegetables and less rice on a new voyage with the ship Tsukuba that was undertaken the following year. On this voyage there were only 14 cases of beriberi and no fatalities. These findings prompted the Japanese Navy to change its staple diet. More barley was used instead of rice, with a drastic reduction of beriberi as a result. However, the physicians of the time concluded that it was not the different diet that was responsible but the improved hygiene. During the Russian-Japanese war of 1904-1905, no fewer than 90,000 cases of beriberi were diagnosed in Japanese soldiers.

The disease occurred in communities that ate white rice, but not in all individuals and the disorder was also seen (to a lesser extent) outside rice-growing areas. The Dutch doctor Christian Eijkman, who won the Nobel Prize in 1929, was working in Indonesia and he used chickens as an animal model for beriberi. After investigating infectious and toxic hypotheses and studying the processing of rice, he established that bran has a protective and curative effect. Bran is a tiny covering membrane that entirely encloses brown rice. It comprises several thin layers. On the outside of the kernel is the fused testa-pericarp (seed coat and fruit wall) and immediately below is the aleurone layer, which is rich in fat and protein. This layer plays an important role in the germination of rice. When an intact grain of rice is exposed to a moist environment, the central core of the grain (embryo) absorbs water. As a consequence, the embryo secretes a plant hormone (gibberellin) that diffuses into the aleurone layer. This layer subsequently secretes amylase, which converts the starch in the endosperm („the grain") into sugars that can then be absorbed by the embryo. The endosperm is rich in starch but poor in thiamine and other compounds. The embryo and the bran, on the other hand, are rich in proteins, fats and thiamine. In white rice the bran and embryo have been removed, as a result of which the rice becomes rancid less quickly but is also deficient in thiamine. When brown rice is steeped in water and partly cooked (parboiled) before preparation, the thiamine in the aleurone layer is able to diffuse into the starchy endosperm. When the rice is then polished, the grain still contains some of the vitamin. This is why beriberi was absent in those regions where the people ate parboiled rice. The Polish researcher Casimir Funk isolated the antiberiberi factor and established that it was an amine. He coined the term „vitamin" for „vital amine". As a result of his discovery, research into deficiency diseases gained momentum. It wasn't until 1936, however, that the correct chemical structure of the antiberiberi factor was finally revealed.

2.4 Beriberi, Rice

Rice plays a central role in the history of beriberi. After all, beriberi occurred chiefly in some regions where rice was the principal diet but not in all such regions. The name „rice" refers to semi-aquatic grasses, mainly Oryza sativa, which originated in Asia. This plant has two major subspecies. Japonica rice grows in slightly colder regions and after preparation the grains are sticky. The tropical, long-grain indica variety has drier, non-sticky grains. African rice is also known as Oryza glaberrima. Wild rice comprises Zizania aquatica and Z. texana, both from the New World. Wild rice is not discussed here. Many rice varieties grow well in shallow water where they have less competition from weeds (paddy rice). The rice plants have specialized roots with many air ducts (aerenchyma), which enable them to live in an anaerobic environment. The epidermis of the roots allows no diffusion of oxygen, as a result of which there is no loss of gas to the water. Some rice varieties grow on dry land (upland rice), provided that the annual rainfall is sufficient (150-200 cm/year).

How is rice harvested and processed?

When harvesting is done by hand, the stalks of the ripe rice are cut with a sickle, gathered into sheaves to dry and then threshed. During the threshing process the grains are released from the stalks and from the surrounding chaff. The chaff consists of protective leathery structures like the awn, palea, lemma and rachilla. In japonica rice the chaff also contains rudimentary glumes. Afterwards the chaff is separated from the grain by winnowing: the mixture is tossed into the air, the heavier grains fall down and the lighter chaff is blown away by the wind. After this treatment the grains are still enclosed by a thin membrane. Intact rice like this, complete with husk and embryo, is called brown whole-grain brown rice. Brown rice may be eaten but it soon becomes rancid due to oxidation of fats in the embryo and thin covering membrane. In some regions brown rice is steeped in water for 12 to 48 hours, drained and then steamed (parboiled rice). This makes it easier to remove the husk but a lot of people don't like the rather musty taste that this treatment gives the rice. Traditionally this thin membrane is removed without parboiling by mechanical polishing, beating or shaking. In this process the embryo is also mechanically removed. The embryo is the tiny structure from which the stalk and roots of a new plant develop. The embryo consists of several parts: the scutellum, epiblast and plumule. After this mechanical process the grains are winnowed again in order to separate the bran and embryos from the grains of rice. This produces white, polished rice. Rice without embryo does have a long shelf stability. Rice must be stored in a dry place. With a humidity higher than 15% the rice will spoil fairly quickly. Lastly, white rice is often mixed with a small amount of talcum powder or chalk to give it a shiny appearance. Rice is seldom milled like wheat or ground into groats.

- Paddy rice or rough rice: the chaff is still present, which makes a 20% difference in weight.

- Brown cargo rice: chaff removed, husk still present. Contains 0.4 mg thiamine per 100 grams.
- Parboiled rice: brown rice steeped and then steamed and hulled. Some of the thiamine penetrates inside the endosperm.
- White peeled polished rice: the chaff and the husk (bran with aleurone layer) as well as the embryo are removed without steaming. Contains 0.04 mg thiamine per 100 grams (i.e. exceptionally little).

White rice can be prepared in various ways. It can be boiled in a copious amount of water, after which the excess water is drained off. Alternatively, white rice can be boiled in a small, precisely measured volume of water, which results in all the water being absorbed. Afterwards it is briefly steamed to prevent the rice from burning or sticking to the pan.

2.5 Beriberi, thiamine deficiency

The biological half-life of thiamine is 9 to 18 days. A biochemical deficiency can become apparent rather quickly, even after just 7 days. The course of the disease is usually somewhat slower. Deficiency may develop in alcoholics, elderly people, malabsorption, use of diuretics, prolonged administration of antacids, dialysis, folate deficiency, diets with a high content of refined grain products and ingestion of thiaminase-containing food. With a deficient diet, clinical complaints often develop in strong young males (high glucose metabolism). Increased thiamine consumption may develop in seriously ill patients, hyperthyroidism, pregnancy, lactation and fever. Chronic malabsorption (chronic diarrhoea) leads to reduced uptake. Serious liver disease may lead to reduced usage. In the clinical context, particular attention should be paid when people are at risk of deficiency and are temporarily receiving no food (persistent vomiting, hyperemesis gravidarum). Especially when a glucose solution is administered quickly by intravenous injection and the metabolism suddenly has to cope with additional substrate, symptoms of acute deficiency may be induced. In practice such a situation can arise when a confused alcoholic with suspected hypoglycaemia is admitted to hospital and a sudden deterioration of the clinical condition is observed after glucose administration.

2.6 Beriberi, clinical aspects

Deficiency signs may initially be very limited. Muscular cramps and paraesthesia may develop. In more severe deficiencies, cardiovascular problems may develop (wet beriberi, Jap.: "shoshin-kakke"). This concerns a high-output heart failure with peripheral pitting oedema, low peripheral resistance, warm extremities, full pulse, "pistol shot" heart tones, swollen neck veins, slight cyanosis and lactate acidosis. When neurological symptoms are prominent, this is called „dry beriberi". This term indicates a mixed motor-sensory neuropathy with pain, paraesthesia and hyporeflexia. Nocturnal muscular pain in the calves may develop. The symptoms are more pronounced in the legs than in the arms. Frequently the patient is unable to get up from the squatting position without assistance. This can resemble thyroid myopathy, but on closer examination, the difference is readily apparent. Acute Wernicke"s syndrome may occur, manifested clinically by horizontal nystagmus, ophthalmoplegia, fever (dysfunction of the hypothalamus), ataxia, confusion and coma. Frequently there are autonomous disorders, both sympathetic hyperactivity with tremor and agitation and hypo activity with hypothermia and low blood pressure. Acute cerebellar ataxia may develop. During alcohol abstinence with simultaneous thiamine deficiency an acute delirium tremens may develop. Retrograde amnesia, confabulation, psychosis and learning difficulties are signs of Korsakoff"s syndrome (psychosis). This develops in 80% of Wernicke patients but it may also have other causes (thalamus haemorrhage or neoplasia). Infantile beriberi is manifested by aphonia, areflexia and heart failure. Breast-fed babies of thiamine-deficient mothers become restless between 2 and 5 months of age, cry frequently and have little appetite. They soon become debilitated and cry soundlessly. They look slightly bloated and present with slight cyanosis and tachycardia. Administration of thiamine IV results in very rapid recovery, often with noticeable improvement in less than 24 hours.

2.7 Beriberi, diagnosis and treatment

The diagnosis of thiamine deficiency is in the first place a clinical one. The clinical suspicion may be confirmed by measuring the erythrocyte transketolase activity in peripheral blood. However, this cannot be performed in all laboratories. Lactate and pyruvate levels in peripheral blood increase. A practical and easy parameter to determine the thiamine status does not exist. Since the vitamin is cheap and not toxic, in case of doubt it is better to administer it. In acute situations a dose of 100 mg thiamine is administered IV. It is best to add 2 ml of a 50% magnesium sulphate solution, since magnesium is a cofactor for transketolase and associated hypomagnesaemia is frequently observed. The clinical response in heart failure is usually very dramatic and fast. Improvement can already be observed just a few hours after administration. The patient is subsequently treated with 20 mg thiamine daily together with a polyvitamin preparation and efforts are made to eliminate the cause of the deficiency (diet, including avoidance of thiaminases, treatment of alcoholism, absorption problems, anti-emetics, etc.). Central lesions usually do not fully recover. In the case of peripheral neural lesions, the degree of recuperation depends upon the duration and severity of the damage.

2.8 Beriberi, prophylaxis

A balanced diet, sufficiently rich in vitamins, is essential. Food supplements may be given to high- risk groups. An unbalanced diet (e.g. based on polished rice) should be avoided. Lactating mothers in endemic regions should preferably take thiamine.

Chapter 3 Pellagra

3.1 Pellagra, Summary

- Disease caused by lack of vitamin PP (niacin) or tryptophan.
- Chiefly in alcoholics and people with an unbalanced diet such as maize.
- Clinical signs: mucositis, dermatitis, diarrhoea and neurological disorders.
- Treatment by nicotinamide supplements and a balanced diet.

3.2 Pellagra, General

For many years, chiefly in regions where maize is the staple diet, a condition has been known which was characterized by cutaneous, mucosal and neurological abnormalities. This condition is known as pellagra. The disease derives its name from an old Italian description. It had been established that prisoners on a prolonged diet consisting solely of maize developed a skin problem. Pelle agra ("pelle", "skin"; "agra", rough). In the 18th century the inexpensive polenta, based on maize meal, was a staple of many rural regions of Italy. It was initially thought that the disease was caused by a fungal toxin in the food. In 1796, Dr Casper Casal, of Oviedo (Spain), described the disease mal de la rosa. The illustration in his work shows manifest skin lesions of the neck. Since that time, this symptom has been known as Casal"s necklace. In the early 20th century, pellagra was a major problem among the poor Southerners of the USA. The work of the American scientist Joseph Goldberger represented a milestone in the history of epidemiology when he discovered that orphans whose diet consisted mainly of maize with molasses developed pellagra and that others (who had a more varied diet) were not affected by the disease. None of the staff ever contracted the disease (they had the first choice of the food). He injected himself and several volunteers with blood from pellagra patients. Not one of them developed the disease. Even eating faecal matter of the patients (!) was likewise unable to induce the disease in these intrepid volunteers, which was a strong argument against an infectious origin. After milk, eggs and meat were put on the menu of the orphanages, pellagra disappeared. A controlled experiment at a State Prison Farm in Mississippi manifestly demonstrated that pellagra only develops after living on an unbalanced diet. An animal model was developed using dogs that were fed on maize and subsequently developed so-called „black-tongue". In 1937, Conrad A. Elvehjem, an agricultural chemist at the University of Wisconsin, discovered that nicotinic acid cures black tongue. It was discovered that the disease has its origins in a deficiency of a compound present in small quantities in food. The compound was designated as vitamin PP (pellagra preventing factor). Sometimes the term vitamin B3 is used. The identification of pellagra as a deficiency disease was not evident. There were sometimes apparently contradictory data. Early in the 20th century, for instance, pellagra was rife in the maize-eating population of Romania. Paradoxically, however, their maize contained more niacin than the food of the indigent population of India, where pellagra did not occur. The explanation was only discovered later when it became clear that maize contained very little tryptophan and that much of the niacin in maize is present as a bound form called niacytin (which is not absorbed in the intestine). The reason why pellagra did not occur in the indigenous maize-eating population of Central America was found to be based on the fact that they used alkali in the preparation of their maize meal, which released niacin from niacytin. They also had a more varied diet, which included a lot of beans (i.e. another food that contains niacin).

3.3 Pellagra, Niacin

Niacin is also known as nicotinic acid, although the latter term is avoided in order not to evoke an association with tobacco and thus make people suspicious. The amide is likewise active (nicotinamide). Niacin is absorbed from food in the stomach and small intestine. A small quantity of niacin is produced endogenously from tryptophan, an essential amino acid. Food that is rich in tryptophan and deficient in niacin will not give rise to clinically manifest deficiency. Alcoholics and people with hyperthyroidism are at higher risk of contracting pellagra. The conversion from tryptophan to niacin is more difficult in people with vitamin B2 (riboflavin) and B6 (pyridoxine) deficiency.

Niacin is required for adequate cellular function and metabolism as an essential component of nicotinamide adenine dinucleotide (NAD) and nicotinamide adenine dinucleotide phosphate (NADP). These compounds are important coenzymes for glycolysis, protein and amino acid metabolism, pyruvate metabolism, pentose biosynthesis, generation of high-energy phosphate bonds, glycerol metabolism, and fatty acid metabolism. In case of deficiency, all sorts of cell functions become deranged.

3.4 Pellagra, Aetiology

On average, a person needs approximately 15 mg niacin on a daily basis. Pellagra may be caused by niacin and/or tryptophan deficiency in the diet. A generally poor balance of amino acids in the diet could also give rise to pellagra. For instance, pellagra frequently affects people who eat sorghum (millet) as a staple food. This grain crop contains high concentrations of leucine. Although this grain contains adequate tryptophan, excessive concentrations of leucine interfere with tryptophan metabolism and subsequent niacin synthesis. Maize (=corn), which is the staple food in many parts of the world, contains very small amounts of tryptophan. Niacin in maize is chemically bound and is not absorbed in the intestine unless the food is treated with alkali. An example of the latter is the tortilla. Food products that contain large quantities of niacin are liver, kidney and yeast and, to a lesser extent, wheat and green vegetables. The bioavailability of niacin from meat, milk, beans and eggs is excellent.

Secondary deficiency may develop in persistent chronic diarrhoea with malabsorption, liver cirrhosis and alcoholism and in the event of prolonged parenteral nutrition being given without vitamin supplements. During treatment with isoniazid (INH) the drug is substituted for nicotinamide in the synthesis of NAD. The resulting molecule is inactive. In prolonged treatment with INH (tuberculosis) it is possible for iatrogenic induced pellagra to be provoked. There are also several situations where tryptophan metabolism is disrupted. For instance, pellagra may develop in carcinoid syndrome, due to the conversion of tryptophan into serotonin (5-hydroxytryptamine). Pellagra also occurs in Hartnup"s disease, an autosomal recessive metabolic disorder associated with defective renal tubular resorption of neutral amino acids. Furthermore, there is a disturbed intestinal absorption that leads to degradation of tryptophan in the intestine. The clinical picture is characterized by a pellagra-like skin rash and cerebellar ataxia. In AIDS-patients, tryptophan metabolism is disturbed (low levels of tryptophan in plasma), but this does not lead to pellagra.

3.5 Pellagra, Clinical Aspects

Clinically, the disease is identified by the so-called classical three Ds: dermatitis, diarrhoea and dementia. Mucositis should also be added to these characteristic symptoms. The symptoms may develop alone or in combination. Several types of skin lesions are recognized. Patients initially present with erythematous skin lesions followed by vesicles, bullae, crusting and desquamation. Secondary infection may develop, including wound myiasis. These fairly rapid developing symptoms are located on parts of the body that are usually exposed to the sun and on trauma sites. The most conspicuous is a sharply defined symmetrical, desquamating rash in the neck area

(Casal"s necklace) and on the forearms. A butterfly-shaped rash may appear on the face, which must be distinguished from skin abnormalities in SLE patients. These skin lesions may be associated with acute intertrigo with erythema, maceration and abrasion; surinfection may develop in the predilection areas (folds of the groin, genitals). In persistent lesions the skin may become thick and rough. Deep cracks or fissures and hyperpigmentation may develop. The lesions resemble those of cutaneous porphyria. Lastly, the lesions may become atrophic, with a dry, scaly and inelastic skin. Pellagra sometimes occurs without skin lesions (pellagra sine pellagra).

Mucositis develops in the mouth, vagina and urethra. A red tongue and stomatitis are characteristic of acute deficiency. The tip and edges of the tongue are the first to be affected. This is followed by a generalized painful, burning glossitis, with swelling of the tongue and hyper salivation. Lip and tongue ulcers may develop. The area around the parotid duct orifice may become necrotic (the area opposite the molar teeth). Deeper mucosae may be affected, with sore throat, oesophageal damage with dysphagia, and abdominal pain. Some patients report loose stools but these complaints are not usually predominant. Caution: chronic malabsorption in itself may induce niacin deficiency. Gastrointestinal hyperaemia, ulceration and proctitis may lead to bloody diarrhoea. When angular stomatitis is present, this usually indicates an associated riboflavin deficiency (vitamin B2).

Neurological symptoms are due to an organic encephalopathy. Psychosis may occur with sleep and memory disorders, anxiety, agitation, rapid irritability, disorientation, confusion and confabulation (compare this with Wernicke-Korsakoff"s syndrome in thiamine deficiency). Mania, delirium, paranoia and depression occur in later stages of the disease. At one time, many pellagra patients were incarcerated in mental institutions. Muscular rigidity may develop together with a cogwheel phenomenon, hyperreflexia and a positive Babinski's sign. In the motor cortex, lysis of Betz's cells and, to a lesser extent, lysis of Purkinje's cells are found. In the spinal cord, the posterior columns are chiefly affected (proprioception tracts; cfr vitamin B12 deficiency). In peripheral nerves there is myelin degeneration, but to what extent this overlaps with the findings in beriberi is unclear (nutritional deficiencies are often mixed). Post-mortem examination may reveal cardiac, adrenal gland, liver and spleen atrophy.

3.6 Pellagra, Diagnosis

When all symptoms and signs are present, the clinical diagnosis is simple. In most cases, however, there are only a few symptoms present. The diagnosis is confirmed by measuring the urinary excretion of N´-methyl nicotinamide (NMN). NMN excretion of <0.8 mg/day suggests niacin deficiency. Patients with pellagra also have increased urinary excretion of coproporphyrins. In clinical practice, a successful test-therapy will confirm the original diagnosis.

Diagnosis of Hartnup"s disease is confirmed by the specific pattern of aminoaciduria in these children.

3.7 Pellagra, Treatment

As there is seldom a deficiency of only one vitamin, treatment should obviously include a polyvitamin preparation in addition to a balanced diet. Specifically, for pellagra, nicotinamide (precursor of niacin) is given as a supplement in a dose ranging from 300 to 1000 mg daily using divided doses. If niacin itself were to be administered, the patient would complain of flushing, paraesthesia and a burning sensation. If no oral supplement can be given (severe stomatitis, severe diarrhoea, uncooperative patient), 100 to 250 mg can be injected SC twice daily. A rapid improvement of the skin lesions and the general condition is usually seen. Neurological improvement is rather slow. A balanced diet is essential for prophylaxis. In some countries flour is systematically enriched with extra niacin.

Note:

High dose of nicotinic acid is used in some cases for the treatment of hyperlipidaemia, but since the development of fibrates and statins this treatment has become obsolete.

Chapter 4 Scurvy

4.1 Scurvy, Summary

- A deficiency of ascorbic acid leads to poor quality collagen.
- Haemorrhages and bone abnormalities dominate the clinical picture.
- Rapid improvement with vitamin C tablets or fresh fruit and vegetables.

4.2 Scurvy, General

Scurvy is a disease caused by lack of vitamin C. The condition was a common ailment aboard European seagoing ships in the early days of world exploration and was a serious problem on long voyages. In 1498, Vasco da Gama lost no fewer than 100 of his original crew of 160 to scurvy. In Magellan's expedition to the Philippines (1519) he lost 200 of his original crew of 218. On board the ships there was a systematic lack of fresh fruit and vegetables. Nowadays, scurvy only occurs in the event of an unbalanced diet with nutritional deficiency, as in some elderly people and alcoholics. Scurvy is sometimes seen in persistent problematical situations in the tropics (refugees, starvation), certainly in warm and dry regions where there is a lack of fresh fruit and vegetables. In the general population living in stable conditions, scurvy is rare.

4.3 Scurvy, Ascorbic Acid

For a long time, the origin of scurvy was a mystery. Before vitamin C was identified, however, a form of empirical treatment and prophylaxis had been discovered, but the nature of the compound that cured scurvy was not clear. A breakthrough came with the discovery that guinea pigs could develop scurvy (guinea pigs, primates and humans – unlike most mammals – are unable to synthesize ascorbic acid). Scientists now had an animal model and an in vivo assay for measuring the antiscorbutic activity of different food products. It was demonstrated that drying, cooking and prolonged exposure to air destroyed the active ingredient. During his research at Cambridge University in 1928, the Hungarian biochemist Szent-Gyorgyi isolated vitamin C. He isolated the compound from adrenal cortex, oranges and cabbage. He received the Nobel Prize for Medicine in 1937. Subsequently it became evident that vitamin C occurs in numerous food products. Vegetables such as broccoli and tomatoes, but also potatoes and citrus fruit have large concentrations of vitamin C. Sir Walter Norman Haworth discovered an efficient synthesis method for the preparation of vitamin C based on a carbohydrate precursor. Sir Norman

Haworth and Paul Karrer (Switzerland) were jointly awarded the Nobel Prize for Chemistry for their work in 1937.

Vitamin C is also known as ascorbic acid. This name refers to „antiscorbutic" (from the Low German term for scurvy: schorbock). Vitamin C is essential for the production of collagen. It is a highly reducing compound and is capable of undergoing reversible oxidation. In consequence, it fulfils a role in redox reactions in the body. Vitamin C promotes the uptake of iron in the intestine and protects folic acid reductase. Vitamin C regenerates antioxidants such as vitamin E, flavonoids and glutathione. It plays a role in the synthesis of steroids and the production of carnitine. The highest concentrations are found in white blood cells, the lens and the brain. The total body pool of vitamin C is approximately 1500 mg. The excess is excreted. There is a turnover of 3% per day, which gives a half-life of approximately 18 days. This explains the latency period for symptoms to occur after starting a diet without vitamin C.

4.4 Scurvy, Collagen

The symptoms of scurvy can be traced back to defective collagen. Collagen is the commonest protein in the animal kingdom. Large amounts of unusual amino acids are found in collagen: hydroxyl sine and hydroxyproline. These are essential for the chemical stability of collagen. The conversion of proline into hydroxyproline is stimulated by the enzyme proline hydroxylase. For this purpose, it uses a Fe^{2+} ion, which is converted during the reaction into Fe^{3+}. This inactivates the enzyme. Enzyme regeneration takes place by an interaction with ascorbate, in which vitamin C is converted into dehydroascorbic acid. For a better understanding of scurvy, we briefly sketch the normal production of the commonest form of collagen. Individual collagen polypeptide chains are synthesized on the ribosomes of the rough endoplasmatic reticulum. The strands are released in the lumen of the endoplasmic reticulum as large precursor molecules, the so-called pro-alpha chains. Signal peptides are still present at front and rear. In the lumen, selected proline and lysine residues are hydroxylized to hydroxyproline and hydroxylysine. Every pro-alpha chain subsequently combines with two other chains to form a triple-strand helix via hydrogen bridges, the fibrillar procollagen. This is subsequently secreted. Procollagen is converted extracellularly into tropocollagen by enzymatic cleavage (with the exception of collagen IV in the basal lamina). Tropocollagen subsequently develops further into mature collagen. Normal collagen is broken down slowly by extracellular collagenases. In scurvy, defective pro-alpha chains are formed (the formation of hydroxy-amino acids is disrupted). They do not form a triple helix and are quickly degraded. The consequences are first noticed first in the tissues where collagen turnover is fastest, such as blood vessels. Owing to the gradual loss of the existing collagen, the blood vessels become progressively fragile.

The hydroxylation of lysine in collagen has a different function than the hydroxylation of proline. It is needed for an unusual form of lysine-crosslinking (covalent intra- and intermolecular crosslinks between modified lysine sidechains). Lysine and hydroxylysine are first deaminated by lysyl oxidase, thereby creating highly reactive aldehyde groups. These groups spontaneously form covalent bonds with one another. Compare this with the pathology in osteolathyrism.

4.5 Scurvy, Aetiology

Primary deficiency is due to an unbalanced diet, i.e. a diet containing less than 10 mg vitamin C per day. Pregnancy, lactation, smoking, surgical procedures, thyrotoxicosis, burns and chronic inflammation increase the body's requirements up to 70-90 mg/day. In achlorhydria and chronic diarrhoea, less vitamin C is absorbed. Ascorbic acid is unstable in the presence of heat and prolonged cooking of food considerably reduces the quantity of active vitamin C.

4.6 Scurvy, Clinical Aspects

A pronounced lack of vitamin C results in a clinical disease known as scurvy. Haemorrhagic problems and bone abnormalities are the most characteristic and recognizable features of this disease. When a diet is chronically deficient in vitamin C (less than 10 mg/day) the first signs may be expected to appear after 3 to 6 months (half-life of vitamin C is about 18 days). This explain why scurvy only appeared on board ships during long sea voyages. The patient first complains of general debility of slow onset, irritability, weight loss and vague muscular and joint pain. Sometimes the first symptom is stiffness in the calves, due to local haemorrhages. Because of the pain in the legs, children may present with pseudo paralysis. In many cases they spontaneously adopt an antalgic posture, with endorotation and bent knees and hips. This is usually seen in babies born prematurely when they reach about 6-12 months of age if they have been fed deficient artificial food. Splinter haemorrhages beneath the fingernails may occur, as in endocarditis. Haemorrhages around the eyes, ears, neck and on the roof of the mouth may occur. are very suggestive of scurvy. Spontaneous bleeding may occur anywhere in the body, including bleeding leading to palpable sub periosteal haemorrhages. Hyperkeratotic hair follicles and perifollicular petechiae (scorbutic purpura) are quasi pathognomonic. Old scars break open. New wounds do not heal or heal poorly. The gums become swollen, purple and spongy and bleed easily. Often there will be secondary infection. In advanced scurvy, teeth fall out spontaneously. Endochondral bone development ceases because osteoblasts no longer produce osteoid. A fibrous area is formed between diaphysis and epiphysis. The costochondral junctions enlarge. This is clinically palpable as a scorbutic rosary (not to be confused with rachitic rosary). Other symptoms include femoral neuropathy and oedema of the legs. Microcytic hypochromic anaemia may develop, which only improves after administration of vitamin C. If other deficiencies are simultaneously present (e.g. folic acid), the anaemia may be macrocytic.

4.7 Scurvy, Differential Diagnosis

Scorbutic rosary on the thorax and bone abnormalities must be distinguished from rachitic rosary (vitamin D deficiency). Scorbutic gingivitis must be distinguished from other causes, such as candidiasis, herpes, trench mouth, syphilis, pemphigus and Behest's syndrome. Scorbutic haemorrhages must be distinguished from other bleeding diatheses. Subperiostal haemorrhage with periost elevation should be distinguished from congenital syphilis.

4.8 Scurvy, Diagnosis

The vitamin C content in peripheral blood can be measured in specialized laboratories. A level of less than 11 µmol/litre is diagnostic for scurvy. Measurement in leukocytes is more precise. The urinary excretion after administration of a test dose of vitamin C can also be measured. A capillary fragility test will be positive. When this is measured using the sphygmomanometer, it is called the Hess capillary test. The regular haemostasis parameters (platelets, coagulation times) are normal. On X-rays of the legs, a „ground-glass" appearance of the epiphysis is often described.

4.9 Scurvy, Treatment

4.9.1 Treatment: Historical Note

Various therapies were used in ancient times but as long as the cause remained unknown, no rational treatment could be suggested. Some people believed that certain plants could be used as a remedy for scurvy. For instance, Cochlearia officinalis (Family: Cruciferae) is known as common scurvy grass. Naval surgeon James Lind was on board the Centurion, a British gunship which had been put to sea in 1740 in order to give a hard time to the Spanish. After three years he had gained considerable experience with scurvy. In 1747, he conducted a kind of clinical trial ahead of its time. He had 12 patients with scurvy on board. They were divided into six groups and each group received a different treatment: (1) one glass of cider a day, (2) 25 drops of an elixir of vitriol three times a day, (3) two spoonsful of vinegar three times a day, (4) half a pint of sea water three times a day, (5) a mixture of garlic, mustard, horseradish and balsam of Peru three times a day, (6) two oranges and a lemon each day. The two men who were given citrus fruit made a spectacular recovery. Cider also brought some improvement, although to a more limited extent. Lind published his findings. In July 1772, Captain Cook set out from Plymouth on board HMS Resolution on an expedition that was to last three years. He didn't lose a single member of the crew to scurvy. A paper that he presented on the prevention of scurvy won for Cook the Royal Society's Copley Gold Medal. He ordered the crew to eat sauerkraut twice a week and gave a malt potion and an orange and lemon to everyone who showed the first signs of scurvy. Furthermore, he made sure that the ship was provisioned with fresh fruit and vegetables each time they made landfall. He also demanded strict hygiene on board, which was very unusual at the time. The Royal Navy implemented Captain Cook's regimen regarding hygiene and ordered that on voyages lasting longer than two weeks, everyone on board was to be given a spoonful of lemon juice and sugar each day. This mixture was incorrectly described as „lime juice", and to this day, British sailors are known as „Limeys". Unfortunately, limes (Citrus medica var acidum) were sometimes used instead of lemons (Citrus medica var limonum). Limes contain much less vitamin C than lemons so that fatalities sometimes occurred and the use of lemon juice was regarded with suspicion. After 1860, only lemons were officially allowed for antiscorbutic use. The reason why scurvy was banished from the long-distance sailing ships of the Chinese Ming dynasty (1368-1644) was due to the fact that the crew were regularly given fresh, germinated soya beans to eat, as part of their traditional food. Unlike non-germinated seeds, these shoots are rich in vitamin C. The importance of the absence of scurvy is not to be underestimated, since the voyages of the Chinese admiral Zheng He (1421) led to world maps, which were obtained by the Portuguese crown and were a crucial element for the major discovery expeditions of Henry the Navigator, opening the world for the West, a fundamental turning point in history.

4.9.2 Treatment: Current Practice

The treatment of scurvy consists of administering extra vitamin C (at least 100 mg three times daily for two weeks) and adjusting the daily diet. Clinical improvement may be expected within one to two weeks. Chronic gingivitis and extensive subcutaneous haemorrhages take a little longer to heal. Vitamin C is sometimes used in Chédiak-Higashi syndrome and in osteogenesis imperfecta. High doses of vitamin C may induce haemolysis in G6PD deficiency. At such high doses, false positive results may be obtained for occult blood in stools (guaiac test).

4.10 Scurvy, Prophylaxis

A sufficiently varied diet containing fruit and green vegetables will prevent the development of scurvy. The systematic, prolonged cooking of all food should be avoided. Vitamin C 60-100 mg/day PO provides protection against scurvy. Some people use vitamin C mega doses in the hope of preventing colds and other ailments. There is little evidence to support this but no definitive conclusion has yet been reached. Urinary acidification does, however, occur. Vitamin C is metabolized to oxalate. When mega doses vitamin C are consumed on a daily basis, this might facilitate the formation of oxalate kidney stones but there is no consensus on this.

Chapter 5 Rickets - Osteomalacia

5.1 Rickets - Osteomalacia, Summary

- Vitamin D in food: sequentially converted in the skin (sunlight), liver and kidneys
- Calcitriol needed for mineralization of osteoid and calcium uptake in the intestine
- Deficiency in children (epiphyseal plate still open) leads to rickets.
- Deficiency in adults (epiphyseal plate closed) leads to osteomalacia.
- Irregularly frayed, wide, cup-shaped distal ulna and radius, rachitic rosary, hypocalcaemia.
- Pseudo fractures, bone deformities, gait disturbance.
- Rapid recovery after deficiency correction, except if end-organ resistance.

5.2 Rickets - Osteomalacia, General

Vitamin D is essential for the proper functioning of the human body. Rich sources of vitamin D are oil derived from fish liver (e.g. cod liver oil) and egg yolk. In Europe, milk is enriched with vitamin D. One microgram of vitamin D is equivalent to 40 IU. Overdosing has toxic consequences. Calcium metabolism is fairly complicated: parathormone (PTH), vitamin D, calcitonin, the calcium- phosphorus product and the major calcium buffer in the skeleton all play a role. For details, see physiology and endocrinology textbooks.

5.3 Rickets - Osteomalacia, Nomenclature

The nomenclature of the various molecules is rather complicated. Not all the names are equally important. Here is an overview and brief summary:

Vitamin D	a general term used to designate this group of compounds.
7-dehydrocholesterol:	the endogenous precursor of cholesterol and of vitamin D3.
Ergosterol	provitamin D2 or 7,22-didehydrocholesterol
Lumisterol	an isomer of pre-vitamin D3
Tachysterol	an isomer of pre-vitamin D3
Vitamin D1	a 1:1 mixture of lumisterol (related to Ergosterol) and vitamin D2.
Vitamin D2	ergocalciferol. Synthetically prepared from Ergosterol via UV irradiation.
Vitamin D3	cholecalciferol = calciol
25-OH-D3	Calcidiol
1,25-(OH)2-D3	calcitriol, physiologically the most active
24,25-(OH) 2-D3	non-active compound

5.4 Rickets - Osteomalacia, Metabolic Conversions Of Vitamin D

Vitamin D is present in food as a fat-soluble provitamin. Vitamin D is regarded as a sterol, although the B ring of the molecular steroid squeleton is open. A photochemical conversion and two hydroxylation's take place in the body before the final form is reached. The absorption of vitamin D is determined by the fat content of the food, by the proper functioning of the pancreas (lipase) and by the presence of sufficient bile. After absorption in the intestine, the provitamin is first transported to the skin, where a photochemical conversion takes place via ultraviolet light. Vitamin D3 is thus formed. This compound can also be produced via UVB radiation from an endogenous precursor, 7-dehydrocholesterol or pre-vitamin D3. [Sunlight breaks the B ring of the cholesterol structure to form pre-D3. Pre-D3 then undergoes a thermal induced rearrangement to form D3. Continued irradiation of pre-D3 leads to the reversible formation of lumisterol and Tachysterol which can revert back to pre-D3 in the dark.] Vitamin D3 is subsequently bound to a carrier protein and transported to the liver, where an initial hydroxylation takes place with the formation of 25-OH-D3. In the kidneys, 25-OH-D3 is further hydroxylated to the metabolically much more active form 1,25-(OH)2-D3 (calcitriol). A similar hydroxylation takes place in the placenta. Extra-renal synthesis of 1,25-(OH)2-D3 may occur in pathological conditions, such as sarcoidosis and other granulomatous disorders. In the blood there is approximately 500 times more 25-OH-D3 present than 1,25-(OH)2-D3. The receptor of 1,25-(OH)2-D3 is located in the cytoplasm of the cell. After binding, the complex migrates to the cell nucleus where (as a transcription factor) it mediates the expression of various genes. The most important functions of vitamin D are to promote normal bone formation by mineralization of the osteoid and to maintain calcium homeostasis (together with parathormone and calcitonin).

Diet with provitamin and fat⇒intestine with bile and lipase⇒skin and sunlight⇒liver ⇒kidneys⇒ end organ.

5.5 Rickets – Osteomalacia, Aetiology

Rickets and osteomalacia develop when there is insufficient vitamin D, when its metabolism is disturbed or when the tissues are resistant to its activity (e.g. mutation of the vitamin D receptor). By following the metabolic chain that leads to the active 1,25-(OH)2-D3 the various causes of osteomalacia/rickets can be visualized. For instance, the food may contain too few precursors. If there is insufficient fat in the diet, or there is insufficient bile and the fat is not absorbed (steatorrhea), a deficiency of fat-soluble vitamins (ADEK) will occur. Prolonged treatment with cholestyramine is a risk factor. Insufficient exposure to sunlight is also an aetiological possibility. Dark-skinned people residing for a long time in the northern hemisphere are a high-risk group. This also applies to protective clothing and people who spend most of their time indoors (elderly people and Islamic women and children are high-risk groups). For instance, rickets/osteomalacia is not uncommon in Indian and Pakistani immigrants in Britain. A lack of direct sunlight and calcium (chelation of calcium by the phytates in their traditional diet and low intake of milk) contributes to the problem. Rarely, the conversion of 25-OH-D3 to 1,25-(OH)2-D3 in the liver may be disturbed by a genetic enzyme defect (type 1, genetic vitamin D-resistant rickets). Some anticonvulsants, such as phenobarbital, induce liver enzymes, resulting in the accelerated breakdown of 25-OH-D3. Phenytoin and phenobarbital moreover have an inhibiting effect on calcium absorption in the intestine. There are several diseases that may be associated with vitamin D deficiency, each of which, however, is rare, such as hypoparathyroidism, genetic diseases such as hereditary hypophosphatemia, or vitamin D-resistant rickets. Rarely, osteomalacia develops as a result of certain tumours.

5.6 Rickets - Osteomalacia, Clinical Aspects

Metabolic bone disease caused by vitamin D deficiency is known as rickets in children and as osteomalacia in adults. [NB. Watch out for possible confusion: rickets has nothing to do with rickettsiosis, which is an infectious disease.] These diseases result from common pathogenic factors but differ in their clinical and pathological expression because of the differences between growing and mature bones. In children, the calcification of osteoid in the developing bones is disturbed. The abnormalities are clearest in the areas of most active growth, i.e. the epiphyses. In chronic deficiency there is resorption of trabecular and cortical bone, which is not compensated by mineralisation of osteoid. Adequate treatment with vitamin D causes a rapid reversal of this situation. Normal enchondral bone formation is resumed. In adults, the changes are similar but are not limited to the extremities of the long bones.

Maternal osteomalacia leads to changes in the bones of the foetus and even to tetany in the new born (hypocalcaemia). Young infants with vitamin D deficiency are restless and sleep poorly. They have reduced mineralization of the skull (craniotabes). On the thorax, palpable lumps develop at the costochondral junctions: costochondral beading (rachitic rosary). Harrison's groove, corresponding to the costal insertion of the diaphragm, may be present. In children from 1 to 4 years of age there is an increase in the width of the epiphyseal cartilages at the distal extremities of the tibia, fibula, ulna and radius ("erlenmeyer deformity"). Kyphoscoliosis may develop and walking is delayed. Older children and adolescents experience walking as painful and in extreme cases develop bowlegs or knock-knees.

Bone changes, visible on X-rays, precede clinical signs, becoming evident in the 3rd or 4th month of life – sometimes even at birth if the mother is severely vitamin D deficient. Bone changes in rickets are most evident at the distal ends of the radius and ulna. The bony ends lose their sharp, clear outline. They are cup-shaped and show a spotty or frayed outline. Later, the distance between the ends of the radius and ulna and the metacarpal bones appears to be increased because the noncalcified ends are invisible on the X-ray. As healing begins, a thin white line of calcification appears at the epiphysis, becoming denser and thicker as calcification proceeds.

In adults, osteomalacia occurs, particularly in the vertebrae, pelvis and legs. Fine lines appear in the cortex: ribbon-like areas of demineralization, the so-called pseudo fractures or Looser's lines. Histologically they consist of focal accumulations of non-calcified osteoid. Preferential localizations for pseudo fractures are the lateral edge of the scapula, femur neck, medial femoral shaft, ribs and ramus pubis. Looser's lines are usually symmetrical, extending perpendicularly to the cortex, are manifestly shorter than the diameter of the bone and display no callus formation. As the bones soften, body weight may cause bowing of the long bones, vertical shortening of the vertebrae and flattening of the pelvic bones, which narrows the pelvic outlet. This may subsequently cause difficulties in childbirth.

5.7 Rickets - Osteomalacia, Laboratory Findings

The various vitamin D metabolites are measured in plasma. In healthy people, normal levels for 25-OH-D3 are 25 to 40 ng/mL (62 to 100 nmol/L) and 20 to 45 pg/mL (48 to 108 pmol/L) for 1,25-(OH)2-D3. In nutritional rickets and osteomalacia, 25-OH-D3 levels are very low and 1,25-(OH)2-D3 is undetectable. Hypophosphatemia and high serum alkaline phosphatase are characteristic. Calcaemia is low or normal, depending upon the effectiveness of parathormone (secondary hyperparathyroidism) in restoring serum calcium to normal. In hereditary vitamin D-dependent rickets, laboratory findings vary.

5.8 Rickets - Osteomalacia, Overview

- Causes: Poor diet Fat malabsorption (intestinal or liver problem) Lack of sunlight Chronic renal failure: lack of 1,25-(OH)2-D3 and hyperparathyroidism Chronic renal tubular acidodis (urine is too alkaline for the acidic blood) Accelerated breakdown by liver enzyme inductors Genetic: defect in the metabolic chain or a resistant receptor in the end organ.
- Bone: Incomplete mineralization
  Irregularly frayed and cupping metaphyseal surfaces Bone pain, bowlegs or knock-knees Hypocalcaemia sometimes with tetany in osteomalacia: also loss of cortical bone Pseudo fractures at preferential localizations

5.9 Rickets - Osteomalacia, Differential Diagnosis

A review of the patient's history may suggest nutritional problems. Rickets must be distinguished from scurvy (cf. scorbutic rosary), congenital syphilis (serologic tests) and from chondrodystrophy (large head, short extremities, thick bones; normal Calcaemia, phosphataemia and alkaline phosphatase levels). Osteogenesis imperfecta, cretinism, congenital dislocation of the hip, hydrocephalus and poliomyelitis should be readily distinguishable. Tetany must be distinguished from convulsions due to other causes. Vitamin D-resistant rickets may be caused by severe renal damage, as in chronic renal tubular acidosis (e.g. Fanconi's syndrome or X-linked hypophosphatemia). Osteomalacia must be distinguished from other causes of bone decalcification, such as hyperparathyroidism, senile or postmenopausal osteoporosis, osteoporosis of hyperthyroidism, steroid use, Cushing's syndrome and atrophy of disuse. X-ray findings, hypocalcaemia, high alkaline phosphatase levels and serum vitamin D levels confirm the diagnosis.

5.10 Rickets - Osteomalacia, Treatment

Vitamin D is used to treat rickets, osteomalacia and renal osteodystrophy. The latter is a bone disease that occurs in chronic renal failure and is characterized by a combination of osteomalacia, osteoporosis and secondary hyperparathyroidism. In the treatment of rickets/osteomalacia it is recommended that the Calcaemia be monitored since vitamin D supplements are very potent and can easily induce hypercalcaemia. With adequate calcium and phosphorus intake, and when the disease is caused by dietary deficiency or insufficient exposure to sunlight, treatment usually consists of vitamin D2 (ergocalciferol) or vitamin D3 (cholecalciferol), in addition to dietary advice and light therapy. Rickets and osteomalacia can be treated with vitamin D 0.02-0.1 mg (800-4000 IU)/day for 6 weeks. Serum 25(OH)-D3 and 1,25(OH)2-D3 (calcitriol) levels begin to rise within 48 hours. Phosphataemia rises in about 10 days. After 6 weeks the dose can be reduced to a maintenance level of 10 µg (400 IU)/day. If tetany is present, vitamin D should be supplemented with calcium salts during the first week. Some cases require massive doses. In patients with renal failure the above-mentioned products are not active and alphacalcidol (1-alpha-hydroxyvitamin D3) should be used in preference. This product is converted in the liver into calcitriol, thus eliminating the need for renal metabolization. In patients with massive steatorrhoea, large doses must be used, e.g. 50,000 to 100,000 IU/day PO or 10,000 IU/day IM, together with adequate calcium and sunlight.

Treatment summary:

If dietary deficiency	Calcium tablets with vitamin D (500 IU), 1 to 2 tablets/day
If malabsorption	Parenteral calciferol, 7.5 mg/month
If vitamin D- resistance	Trial therapy with calciferol, 10,000 IU/day PO
If renal osteomalacia	Alfacalcidol, 1 µg/day PO and Calcaemia monitoring

5.11 Rickets - Osteomalacia, Prophylaxis

Disease prevention is based upon health education and efforts must be made to ensure that the communities in question really understand and act on the information provided. Human breast milk is deficient in vitamin D (1.0 µg/L = 40 IU/L), whereas fortified cow's milk contains ten times as much. Breastfed infants should therefore be given a supplement of vitamin D (300 IU)/day) from birth to 6 months, at which time they are given a more diversified diet. In the Far East, a single IM dose of 2.5 mg (100,000 IU) ergocalciferol is sometimes given to adolescents, which offers protection for several months.

5.12 Rickets - Osteomalacia, Vitamin D Intoxication

When accidental or intentional high doses of vitamin D are taken, the clinical picture is dominated by hypercalcaemia. The rate at which the symptoms develop depends upon the dose and duration of excess vitamin D intake. The first symptoms are anorexia, nausea, vomiting, polyuria, polydipsia and pruritus. Polyuria is secondary to a massive increase of urinary calcium excretion. Complications consist of metastatic calcifications (nephrocalcinosis!) and renal failure. Patients sometimes complain of eye irritation. Physical examination may reveal a band like grey-white opacity across the corneal surface: band keratopathy. Treatment consists of stopping further administration of vitamin D and giving corticosteroids. Urinary acidification is recommended. Diuretics serve no useful purpose. Bisphosphonates such as pamidronate (an osteoclast inhibitor) may be used in extreme cases.

Chapter 6 VITAMIN A

6.1 Vitamin A Physiology

6.1.1 Vitamin A and Provitamin A

The term vitamin A should be used as the generic descriptor for retinoids exhibiting the qualitative biological activity of retinol. The main molecular structure contains a cyclic part and a non-cyclic chain with 5 double bonds in the all-trans position. A functional group is found at the end of the non-cyclic part which can be an alcohol (retinol), an aldehyde (reninaldehyde), a palmitate (retinol palmitate), etc. The term provitamin A carotenoid should be used as the generic descriptor for all carotenoids exhibiting qualitatively the biological activity of beta-carotene. In order to have some indicator of activity we now speak of retinol equivalents.

1mcg retinol equivalent	= 1 mcg retinol = 6 mcg beta carotene = 12 mcg other carotenoids
1 IU (international unit)	= 0.3 mcg retinol
1mcg retinol	= 3.3 IU

6.1.2 Metabolism

Vitamin A is, after ingestion, absorbed in the gut in the chylomicron fraction and then transported via the lymphatics, to the liver. The availability of fats in the intestine will influence the fraction of the available vitamin that will be absorbed. Once stored in the liver as retinol palmitate it will be transported to the target organs bound to a protein, the retinol binding protein (RBP). Zinc and an adequate intake of protein are required for normal production of RBP.

6.1.3 Vitamin A Activities

- Function in rhodopsin for night vision.
- Role in the differentiation process of epithelial tissues.
- Necessary for normal ciliary function.
- Role in the synthesis of glycoproteins.
- Stabiliser of lysosomal membranes.
- Function in the cell mediated immunity.
- Reproduction.

As a result of this wide spectrum of activities, a deficit of vitamin A will have several effects.

1. It causes night blindness.

2. It causes Xerophthalmia.

3. Increases the overall mortality. Some authors state by as much as 16%.

4. Increases morbidity. A higher frequency of diarrhoea, ARTI (acute respiratory tract infection) and otitis media have been noted.

5. Is an attributing factor in the causality of stunting.

6.2 Importance of The Problem

1. Vitamin A deficiency is the most important cause of blindness in children in the world today. More important than gonorrhoea, trachoma, cataract, onchocerciasis, trauma or glaucoma.

2. It is an important factor in the cause of stunting which is more prevalent than malnutrition.

3. It is an important contributing factor in mortality which is still very high in the majority of the third world countries. This can for a large extend be explained by the role vitamin A has in maintaining the immunological response and the differentiation and maintenance of epithelial surfaces, like the skin, bronchi, gut and genito-urinal tract, which are more prone to invasion by bacteria in a vitamin deficiency states. These effects are present well before there are overt clinical signs at the level of the eye.

6.3 Diagnosis of Vitamin A Deficiency

6.3.1 Definitions

Before going into further details it is necessary to revise some important definitions:

Xerophthalmia Although it literally means (xeros= dry; ophthalmos = eye) dryness of the eye and is used as such by the ophthalmologists, it is used in a broader sense in the public health context of vitamin A deficiency. Here it means all lesions, internal and external, attributable to the deficit of vit A: dryness of conjunctiva and cornea, Bitot spots, keratomalacia and night blindness.

Keratomalacia Is a liquefaction necrosis of the cornea varying from small ulcerations to softening and rupture of the cornea, with resulting loss of anterior chamber fluid and collapse of the eye. In young children keratomalacia can occur without preceding stages such as dryness of the conjunctiva or Bitot spots.

Xerosis Is a dryness. The clinical dryness of the conjunctivae in vitamin A deficiency is due to squamous metaplasia and keratinization.

Bitot spots Greyish - whitish spot, foamy aspect to be found on the conjunctiva. It can have different forms, round, oval, small spots dispersed. The triangular form is the most frequent. The basis is against the rim of the cornea "the limbus cornea" and the top points to the outside of the eye. Can be uni- or bilateral. This lesion does not hurt.

The diagnosis can be made:

- Clinically
- By measuring hepatic reserves.
- By measuring plasma levels of retinol.
- Impression cytology
- Vital staining

6.3.2 Clinical Picture

The natural course of the disease progresses from night blindness to dryness of the cornea, sometimes with Bitot spots, to keratomalacia. Night blindness is not always perceived because it is a subjective sign on the one hand and because it's perception is very much influenced by the availability of electricity on the other hand.

Night blindness Is the inability to see in poor lighting conditions like those which prevail at the end of the day when the evening is setting, and a longer adaptation of vision to the dark, like when one is getting from a light to a darker environment. People will complain of stumbling over objects in the house in the evening or that their children can't find the parents anymore in the house in the evening. Quantifiable: dark adaptation test, but difficult to evaluate objectively in children.

Conjunctival Xerosis Dry appearance of the cornea, loses it lustre. Some undulation can be seen.

Bitot spots A triangular whitish, pearly coloured spot, which is usually found on the lateral side of the conjunctiva. Has a foamy appearance. Note that the progression of the clinical picture does not always pass through this stage.

Corneal dryness The light reflex of the cornea loses its well-defined appearance and becomes mottled and hazy. The cornea becomes less translucent and more opaque.

Keratomalacia Small lesions like ulcerations can develop. The cornea loses its spherical appearance, softens and bulges. Eventually it ruptures and the anterior chamber liquid runs out and the eye collapses.

Fundus examination Small white spots can be found on the retina. Moderate forms (loss of night vision, conjunctival dryness) will disappear after 2-4 days of treatment without leaving any lesions or sequelae.

Plasma retinol	
>= 30 mcg/100 ml	Normal
30-20 mcg/100 ml	Mild deficiency
20- 10 mcg/100 ml	Associated with night blindness, Bitot spots Moderate deficiency
< 10 mcg/100 ml	Definitely low, severe deficiency

6.3.3 Biochemical Diagnosis

Hepatic reserves Are only measured on an experimental and research basis. Are measured as a rapid dose response (RDR). After administration of a small dose of retinol (1.800 IU) the plasma retinol levels are measured again and compared with the retinol concentrations before the administration. If the concentration increases with more than 20 % we say that the reserves are low.

Plasma levels The problem with measuring plasma retinol levels is that they only change after a prolonged period of vitamin deficit, due to the buffering action of the liver. Their use is limited to research evaluations of vitamin A deficiency and of very little practical use in real life situations.

6.3.4 Impression Cytology

A technique to detect the degree of metaplasia of the conjunctiva. The lack of differentiation and the decrease or absence of goblet cells is looked for. Not a routine diagnostic test.

Vital staining: Detecting the degree of conjunctival metaplasia by putting dye (Lissamon green or Bengal rose) on the conjunctiva. This method lacks specificity.

6.4 Vitamin A Deficiency as a Public Health Problem

Since vitamin A deficiency gives a multitude of signs and symptoms reflecting different degrees of progress a classification has been proposed by the WHO. Minimum prevalence rates for the clinical stages of Xerophthalmia and low plasma retinol levels have been published by the WHO to assist in defining the public health significance of vitamin A in the community.

Criteria for assessing the Public Health Significance of Xerophthalmia and vitamin A deficiency, based on the prevalence among children aged 6 months - 6 years		
Criterion	Classification	Minimum prevalence
Clinical		
Night blindness	XN	1%
Conjunctival dryness	X1A	
Bitot spots	X1B	0.5%
Corneal Xerosis	X2	
Corneal ulceration/Keratomalacia < 1/3	X3A	0.01%
Corneal ulceration/Keratomalacia >= 1/3	X3B	
Scar	X3B	
Fundus	XS	%

	XF	
Biochemical		
Serum retinol less than 10 mcg/100 ml		%

6.5 Causes of Vitamin A Deficiency

Both an insufficient input and an increased need can result in the deficiency.

6.5.1 Insufficient Intake

- Animal sources of vit A: milk - butter - fish oils - liver - meat - egg yolk
- vegetables: green leafy vegetables – carrots
- fruits: mango - papaya
- oils: palm oil

Infections of the gut, malabsorption, worm infestations and particularly giardiasis decrease vitamin A absorption.

6.5.2 Increased Needs

Infections can increase vitamin A demands dramatically. Some investigators even calculated the increase during infections in the order of 3000 IU per day. Particularly children with measles are very likely to develop a very fast progressing Keratomalacia.

6.5.3 PEM

There is a very strong association of vitamin A deficiency with malnutrition. Both are diseases of the poorer layers of the population and of the deprived. They will have an over all lower food intake but particularly of meats and milk products, sources rich in vitamin A, and of oils and fats, which are necessary for the vitamin A absorption. These children will also have more frequent infections, increasing their demands and interfering with the absorption at the level of the gut. Once their serum protein levels decrease like in severe malnutrition the necessary enzymes for absorption and transportation to the target organs will diminish, aggravating further the deficiency.

6.6 Recommended Daily Intakes

Adult	750 mcg
Pregnancy	750 mcg
Breastfeeding	1200 mcg
Children:	
< 1 yr.	300 mcg
1-4 yrs.	250 mcg
4-6 yrs.	300 mcg
7-9 yrs.	400 mcg
10-12 yrs.	575 mcg
13-15 yrs.	725 mcg

6.7 Treatment

The presence of clinical signs of vitamin a deficiency should be considered and emergency. Large and repeated doses are therefore given. Associated illnesses should always be treated.
Who should be treated?
All children with signs of Xerophthalmia.
 The most urgent are those infants with corneal signs.

All suspected cases.
In an endemic zone, all children with PEM and measles.

Children < 1 yr.	Children 1 yr. and above and adults except pregnant women
100.000 IU immediately	200.000 IU immediately
100.000 IU after 24 hrs	200.000 IU after 24 hrs
100.000 IU after 14 days *	200.000 IU after 14 days
* the last dose is mainly to replenish liver stores	

Below one year of below 8 kg the dose is half of what is found in the vitamin a high dosage capsules. These contain 6 drops. Throw away tree drops and give the remainder.

Pregnant women
- Should not receive large doses of vitamin A due to the possible teratogenic effect.
- Smaller doses up to 10.000 IU per day are safe.
- A total dose of 200.000 IU should be aimed at.

Lactating women
- Should receive 200.000 IU in the first month postpartum.
- One month after delivery again smaller doses up to 10.000 IU per day are preferred.
- This because one month after delivery there is the possibility of renewed pregnancy.

6.8 Prophylaxis

"Appropriateness" is a basic premise for vitamin A intervention. Two conditions dictate whether a program, designed to prevent vitamin A deficiency, is appropriate:
1. A substantial segment of the population is "at risk" of developing clinical or biochemical vitamin A deficiency of sufficient severity to be considered of Public Health importance.
2. The problem is serious enough to warrant the diversion of scarce resources toward a program to control vitamin A deficiency versus other preventable diseases or community projects within the country.

Currently vitamin A prophylaxis is approached through one of the three major intervention strategies:

1. A change in diet directed toward achieving a continuous intake of vitamin A rich food,

2. Fortification of an appropriate dietary vehicle with vitamin A or administration of a single, large dose of vitamin A administered on a periodic basis.

6.8.2 Change in Dietary Intake

Different strategies have been applied to increase dietary intake:

- Promotion of breastfeeding. Children entirely breastfed, provided the mother has adequate daily intakes of vitamin A, do not develop vitamin A deficiency in the first six months of life and have a lower prevalence of mild and severe Xerophthalmia during early childhood.
- Nutritional education.
- Income generating programs.
- Kitchen gardening programs.
- Larger scale agricultural programs.

6.8.3 Vitamin A Fortification

Fortification of Mono-sodium Glutamate in the Philippines and of sugar in Guatemala have been highly successful. The success of this type of program depends on the identification of a suitable vehicle, which has to be consumed by all and particularly the population at risk, and in a continuous and constant fashion. Fluctuations between people and in time should be as small as possible. The cost of the program on a national scale is usually high enough to raise the question as to who is going to bear it; the government, the industry or the consumer. Disagreement over this last point have led to the discontinuation of the fortification programs.

6.8.4 Distribution of Large Dose Vitamin A Capsules

Large doses of 200.000 IU are distributed at regular intervals, most frequently every six months. The seasonal distributions, to protect children in the higher prevalence seasons, reduces cost while maintaining the same impact.

Three delivery strategies are possible:

1. The 'medical' or 'therapeutic' approach, which offers treatment to children who present to a health facility with an illness episode. They will be given a dose of vitamin A according to a set of pre- set criteria of high risk of developing vitamin A deficiency.
2. The 'targeted' distribution which covers groups within the larger general target population; e.g., residents of a high prevalence neighbourhood, those attending mother and child health clinics, etc.
3. The 'universal' distribution in which all pre-school children and not pregnant lactating mothers in a prescribed region are dosed at prescribed intervals by single or multipurpose workers in the community.

The logistics, supervision, personnel demand and cost of this type of program are usually very high compared with the money available for general health care in the country. This type of programme costs 4 BF in India and 8 BF in Indonesia per administered dose. Although effective, large dose distribution has been discontinued in a number of countries for these reasons.

6.9 Vitamin A Toxicity

6.9.1 Acute Hypervitaminosis

Ingestion of large dose can give rise to transient signs and symptoms of toxicity, which are self-limiting and completely reversible. No deaths have been reported after the ingestion of the doses used in treatment and prevention.

Common complaints include headaches and bulging fontanel in young children. Nausea, vomiting, dizziness, headaches have been described in adults. Desquamation of the skin, bone pains and hair loss can occur in the following days.

6.9.2 Chronic Hypervitaminosis

Is due to ingestion of large doses on a daily basis. This can lead to hepatitis, cirrhosis, hair loss, dry scaling skin, hyperpigmentation, hyperostosis and bone pains, hepato-splenomegaly and anaemia. It is therefore recommended not to exceed a daily intake of 3000 mcg in children and 7500 mcg in adults.

6.9.3 Teratogenicity

Although teratogenic in animals, a clear correlation between ingestion of large doses of vitamin A and congenital malformations has not been established. However, it is recommended during pregnancy not to give large doses of vitamin A and not to exceed 10.000 IU per day as treatment dose.